# The Secret Language of Cravings

*Uncover The Intelligence Behind Food Cravings And End Your Battle With Overeating Forever*

## Freedom From Overeating
### Book 1

## Alexandra Amor

Copyedit by Jennifer McIntyre
Cover design by Alexandra Amor

Fat Head Publishing
PO Box 916, Ucluelet, BC, Canada V0R 3A0
AlexandraAmor.com

Published in Canada with international distribution

 Created with Vellum

# The Secret Language of Cravings

# Chapter 1

## *The Messenger*

A messenger comes to your door with information that is going to make navigating your life so much easier and more peaceful.

Diet culture tells us to shoot the messenger.

Alternatively, in this book, I'm going to offer you a way to learn to understand what the messenger is trying to tell you.

# Chapter 2

## *What This Book Isn't*

Very quickly, before we get started, I want to make you aware of what this book isn't. This might seem like an odd way to begin, but it's important.

You're likely used to self-help and/or diet books that provide you with rules and structure or guidelines for how the authors of the books think you should do the thing they're teaching. An example might be 'Fifteen ways to get your alligator to walk on a leash.' That book would contain lots of instructions about the specific type of leash to use with your alligator, the best times of day to walk an alligator, and behavior modification tips to prevent it from eating toddlers on your route.

This book is not written in that style.

Let me be completely frank and say I don't now, nor will I ever, have any suggestions for you about what to eat or when to eat or how to prevent yourself from eating when you feel a craving coming on. How many books of that type have you read in the last few years? And how many have worked for you? I'm just guessing, but I'll bet the answer to that second question is zero because if the answer was even 'one,' then you wouldn't be here.

The reason rules and instructions and new-fangled eating plans don't work for most of us when it comes to changing our eating habits is that they circumvent or ignore the innate wisdom that exists within all of us. As paradoxical as it sounds, that wisdom is speaking to us via our cravings. And as we're going to discuss in a future chapter, until that wisdom knows you've heard what it has to say, it's not going to stop communicating with you via your cravings.

Therefore, instead of rules and guidelines about eating, I'm going to offer you *a description of the surprising way your human design works*, how your cravings are an important part of that design, and what those cravings are trying to tell you. As you begin to understand more about the secret language of cravings, you will likely be able to see how this applies in your life. I won't need to tell you what to do about your cravings because once I've described how they work, either you'll know right away what to do or you'll soon have insights about what to do.

Think of it this way: once you know how an umbrella works, from then on you use it when you need to.

When you feel rain on your face, you don't need to check a list of rules telling you whether it's appropriate to use your umbrella or not. Creating a bunch of rules around umbrella use would only complicate a very simple issue.

The same applies here.


Also, the secret language that food cravings are speaking is the same language that cravings for shopping are speaking. Or gambling. Or alcohol. Or binge eating. Any 'over-ing' behavior is whispering the same message that overeating is. So, if you're wrestling with an 'over-ing' behavior other than overeating, you will benefit from the understanding in this book just as much as someone who's trying to resolve an overeating habit. Anytime you see the word 'overeating,' you can substitute your own over-ing word in its place.


And finally, this book is not an indoctrination. There is no dogma here. It is an invitation for you to explore in your own life what I'm pointing toward. Nothing I can tell you will be more helpful to you than examining and leaning into your own experience. Given all the self-help/diet books you've likely read, you've probably gotten really good at putting aside your own wisdom and experience in the name of following the logic of eating plans and willpower. However, when it comes to resolving a long-held, unwanted overeating habit, what creates lasting, irreversible change is the insights that come when we turn toward our own personal wisdom and experience. If you've ever listened to the interviews on my podcast, Unbroken, you'll notice that my guests often mention having profound insights about life—but the interesting thing is, these are never exactly the same insights. Each person's wisdom speaks to them about the things that will have the most impact for *them*.

This is where the power of exploring this understanding lives. And this is one of the things that makes it entirely different from anything you've explored before.

# Chapter 3

## *Louder*

Imagine this: you're walking down the street, minding your own business, when a stranger rushes up to you and starts speaking to you in an urgent tone. Whatever message she's trying to get across is clearly important, but unfortunately you don't speak the language the stranger is speaking. What she's trying to alert you to is that you are gushing blood from a wound you can't see or feel. The stranger can see it, and she is, of course, determined to make sure you know about it; perhaps she is a paramedic or doctor and feels a sworn duty to serve those who are wounded. Maybe she's just a very nice person who wants to help.

You indicate that you don't understand what the stranger is saying so she starts talking louder. But it's still a language you don't speak, so that doesn't help. Now you're starting to think the stranger is perhaps a little mentally unbalanced, so you try to move past her, saying goodbye, averting your eyes, pretending she doesn't exist. The stranger gets louder still. You're getting embarrassed, so you might try to physically push the stranger away, impressing upon her that you're not interested in her message. The stranger gets louder still and more insistent, so much so that you become locked in a battle with her; you're trying desperately to get away and the stranger is just as desperately trying to let you know that she has some information that is critical to your quality of life.

Your food cravings are like this: a stranger who speaks a language you don't happen to speak.

When we don't pay attention to the message that cravings are trying to deliver, they get 'louder,' i.e., they become stronger and more persistent. We innocently view this as a problem. We think that our cravings are becoming more unmanageable. We might even start referring to ourselves as a 'food addict,' feeling like we are broken or unwell because of the noise we're living with from our cravings. We become locked in a battle of wills with cravings; we work harder to suppress the message, and in response, the cravings themselves work harder to get our attention.

We can try all the tactics and strategies we want to try to get rid of that stranger on the street, but she will not budge. She has a sworn duty to serve those who need her help.

# Chapter 4

## *Tsunami Warning*

I jerked awake, my mind on high alert before I was fully conscious. It took me a moment to realize I'd been woken up by a noise. I lay in the dark, under my down duvet, and listened. The fading sound was reminiscent of an air-raid siren, the kind you hear in WWII movies. Entirely different from the urgent screaming of an ambulance or police siren. This was a long, drawn-out wail that rose to a peak, crested like a wave, and then gradually lowered in volume.

My heart seemed to double its beats per minute. I stared at the dark ceiling, waiting, listening.

Nothing. The sound was no longer there.

I reached over and looked at my phone's lock screen. It was just after 4 a.m.

I put the phone down and lay back. The dark ceiling stared at me, impassive. My elevated heart rate began to slow. I took a few deep breaths and genuinely began to wonder if I'd imagined the sound. Maybe whatever I'd been dreaming about had woken me and I'd brought the noise with me into consciousness as I came out of REM sleep.

I took a few long, deep breaths and waited some more. Silence.

Now I was nearly convinced that my dreaming mind had made up the sound. I rolled over onto my side, closed my eyes, pulled the duvet up higher around my neck, snuggled down, and tried to go back to sleep.

WHHHHOOOOOOOOOooooooooo.

My head popped off the pillow. It was real. I wasn't crazy or dreaming. There was an actual siren going off.

I sat up, pulled my glasses on, grabbed my phone again and went immediately to my town's Facebook group, trying to see if anyone else was hearing what I was hearing. They were. It was a tsunami alert.

Some quick scanning in the dark told me that a 7.9 magnitude earthquake had struck off the coast of Alaska and a tsunami alert had been issued for the British Columbia coast where I live, for as far away as California, and for all coastal regions in between.

"Welcome to island life," I thought as I rolled out of bed and began thinking about what I should pack to bring with me to the high-ground gathering place.

. . .

While I didn't exactly enjoy spending the next couple of hours sitting on the cold, hard floor of the high school gymnasium with approximately 400 other sleepy-yet-startled town residents, I did develop a new appreciation for the tsunami warning system the town had in place. I'm slightly embarrassed to say that until that night I didn't realize the system existed. I'd only lived in the town for 11 weeks and was still learning about the community and its wild, natural surroundings.

Ucluelet (pronounced You-clue-let) occupies a rocky, narrow peninsula that is a little more than six square kilometers in size, and juts out into the Pacific Ocean, exposed on the west side to the rolling waves and ferocious storms that pound the shore. And yet, inexplicably, I hadn't been thinking about tsunamis when I moved there. I was perhaps peripherally aware that they could be something I'd encounter, but at the time most of my attention was occupied with grieving the deaths of my mother and my only sibling. It hadn't occurred to me to go to the town's website and get acquainted with the tsunami awareness program.

But it turns out I didn't need to. The sirens were there to alert me. And they did exactly that: waking me out of a deep sleep and letting me know what was happening so that I and the rest of the town could get ourselves to higher ground.

Surprising fact: our food cravings are just like that siren. They are there to help you, not hurt you. They are not a sign that you are broken or flawed or faulty in some way. They are *not* letting you know that you are lazy or lack willpower.

Your cravings are a signal, a sign, an alert. They are part of your perfect human design. I know it doesn't seem that way. Believe me, I know from personal experience that they can seem like a *huge* problem, something to be conquered, eradicated, or, at the very least, managed.

How has that approach worked for you so far?

Not well?

Me too.

But I thought that food-craving management was the only path available to me. I spent 30 years trying to heal, manage, remove, silence, and control my food cravings. I threw every self-help program, healthy diet, structured eating plan, and healing modality at them, spending so much time and goodness only knows how much money, all to no avail. The cravings remained, my weight kept climbing, and my frustration with myself grew.

*Three decades* of giving everything I had to fix a problem, only to have it get worse.

Then, in 2017, a friend introduced me to a field of spiritual psychology called the Three Principles, or the

Inside-Out Understanding, which brought to light the idea that my food cravings weren't, in fact, a problem. I learned that, surprisingly, the cravings were trying to communicate with me and help me. That was when everything changed.

I know it can seem like I'm being flippant or dismissive when I say that your cravings aren't a problem. I remember when I first began learning about this understanding and I'd hear people say this. I'd shake my head and think they were viewing life through very thick rose-colored glasses. Either that or they were deeply deluded. Couldn't they understand how much suffering was involved with a deep-seated overeating habit? Didn't they know how hard I'd worked to change and fix it? But as I listened and learned, gradually I began to see what they were pointing toward. And now I want to point you in the same direction.

Your food cravings are like that tsunami warning siren that woke me up in the wee hours of a cold January morning in 2018: they serve a very important purpose. And just like the siren points us coastal dwellers in the direction of safety, your cravings are pointing you toward your perfect human design, toward a life free of cravings and extra weight. Once you learn the language of the signals, they can then drop away because they're no longer needed—just as, when the tsunami threat has passed, the siren goes quiet.

# Chapter 5

## *About Me*

Before we get too deep into things, let me expand on what I just shared about myself so that you know a little bit about who you're listening to.

As I mentioned, until I was introduced to the field of spiritual psychology that we're exploring in this book I struggled mightily with an unwanted overeating habit. I started to notice what felt like an unhealthy preoccupation with food when I was in my late teens. I found that I was comforting myself with food more often than I thought was healthy for me. I felt I was a little too focused on where my next meal was coming from and what it would be, and it didn't look to me like others were feeling the same way about food. I was a sugar fiend so, for example, when eating out with friends, I would eat the main course simply because it would lead to dessert. If I had been less inclined to be polite, I would have skipped the main course entirely and gone straight for the chocolate cake.

Pretty much as soon as I noticed this stuff going on I began to look for solutions to these thoughts and feelings about food and try to figure out how to 'correct' them. I started going to Weight Watchers in my very early 20s, although I only lasted a few weeks at the meetings. (I would circle back to that program several times over the next 30 years.) Thus began a search for understanding about my own behavior that took me to every self-help book I could get my hands on and every psychology-based strategy for ending an unwanted habit. I tried talk therapy, EMDR, mindfulness, radical self-compassion, EFT (tapping), something called Psych-K, cognitive behavioral therapy (CBT), Byron Katie's The Work, and Rational Recovery, to name but a few. I followed Geneen Roth and read all her books.

I tried very permissive ways of eating and thinking about food, and also very restrictive ones. I hired food coaches and attended classes. I spent a year focused on a program that at the time was called The Solution, attending teleclasses (this was before online classes became a thing) and working my way through weighty textbooks and workbooks. The program cost a couple of thousand dollars and was science based; it was also CBT adjacent, I seem to recall. In the 2010s I dove deep into another CBT-adjacent field called Acceptance and Commitment Therapy; I read all those books too, and practiced what they were preaching.

With the exceptions of prayer, diet pills, and surgery, I tried everything.

None of it made even the smallest dent in my habit. Sometimes for a few days or weeks the habit would fade into the background slightly, but very quickly it would come roaring back and take over my life again.

This cycle went on for 30 years.

There were only so many solutions on offer, so, as I said, I would sometimes circle back around to ones I'd tried before and give them another shot, thinking that somehow I'd missed the message and/or had not understood the teaching and that was why it hadn't worked. At times, I was convinced *I* was the problem, that I was broken and somehow unfixable. The evidence for this was right there; none of the things I'd tried had worked, therefore the issue, I believed, must lie within me. At other times, I decided there must not be a solution to resolving how I felt.

I had periods of giving up, times when I would think, "Forget it. This is too hard and I'm too frustrated." But within days I'd be back in my favorite Vancouver bookstore, scanning the shelves in the diet or habit-breaking sections, looking for a book I hadn't read. Or, when the internet came into being, searching online.

My weight was climbing while all of this was going on, of course, and I was increasingly ashamed about putting so much time, effort, and money into something only to observe zero or negative results. I would share with my close girlfriends every time I found a new approach to try that I was convinced would work, only to fail over and over. It was mortifying. For decades, my day jobs always took a back seat to searching for an answer to this problem, which felt like my real full-time job.

What kept me searching for answers was a deeply rooted and instinctual sense that it had to be possible to be at peace in my relationship with food. I saw other people do it; people who could get up from the table, walk away, and move on to the next thing in their lives, while I was left with an aching, gaping hole inside me that whispered, "There's never enough." That hungry voice was with me at every meal, and often outside mealtimes. None of the strategies and tactics that I'd tried had quieted it even one decibel. And yet, despite decades of failure, I believed it had to be possible to heal that aching void within me and quiet that voice. It was like walking around with a pebble in my shoe all those years; I just knew there had to be a more comfortable way to live.

Then, in 2017, a friend introduced me to the field of spiritual psychology that I'm sharing in this book. At first, I grabbed onto it the way the drowning woman grabs onto a life ring, the same way I'd done with everything else I'd tried. I also initially lumped this understanding in with all the other self-help strategies I'd explored, thinking it was simply a vein in that mine that I hadn't encountered yet. But gradually I began to realize that this was something different. The teachers

I was following kept referring to the idea that I wasn't broken and didn't need fixing. That didn't make sense to me, but I liked the way it sounded so I kept exploring, kept learning. Gradually, understanding coupled with my own insights began to shift things for me. I started to see what they were pointing toward.

And much to my amazement, some of my unwanted eating habits began to fall away on their own. That's when I knew there was something different here, something profound. Now, a few years later, my unwanted eating habits are entirely gone, my weight is falling, and the shame that I lived with about my failure to fix myself has also disappeared. All this happened without willpower, without structured eating plans or programs, without rules about what I should and should not be eating. The fight is over.

The battle that I waged for 30 years and the suffering I endured have prompted me to share what I see and what I have learned. I know I am not alone and that there are others like me whose suffering would be eased by exploring this paradigm known as the Three Principles. I now teach and coach about the principles, and I also host a twice-weekly podcast about this understanding called Unbroken.

If I had a Wikipedia page, it would also share that I'm Canadian. I live on an island off the west coast of British Columbia. My first book was an award-winning memoir about ten years I spent in a cult in Vancouver in the 1990s. (Yes, really.) I love driving and napping, though not usually at the same time. I also love to read and walk on the beaches near my home. My favorite cheese is stinky, gooey Brie. My favorite month is September.

That's probably enough about me. Let's get back to learning the secret language of cravings.

# Chapter 6

## *Why Everything You've Tried Hasn't Worked*

You've probably tried many diets and eating plans and programs in order to curb your overeating habit. Me too. And I'm guessing that all that resulted in was an inability to achieve your goal of stopping your cravings and losing weight. That probably has you feeling like a failure. I did as well.

If there was just one thing you could take away from this book, I'd like it to be this: You are not a failure or a problem. There is nothing wrong with you.

I had a hard time grasping that idea when I first started exploring this understanding. I wondered how people could say that there was nothing wrong with me when the whole reason I was learning about the inside-out nature of life was that I felt so broken. I felt there was so much wrong with me, and that it was reflected in my eating habits and my increasing weight, so how could someone say there was nothing wrong with me? It made no sense. So, I'll explain that statement by saying this: A diamond that is covered in layers of mud is still a diamond.

Instead of you being a failure or a problem, what's wrong is that the understanding we have around how the human psychological experience works is back-wards. The old psychological paradigm that we're used to focuses on the mud around the diamond that is each of us. It suggests that the mud can somehow affect the diamond. It is a paradigm of pathology.

The new psychological paradigm that I'm exploring in this book, and in my work, flips that on its head. It points toward every human being's innate resilience, wisdom, and well-being. It is a paradigm of health. That's the diamond that is underneath the mud. Your health is always there.

Unfortunately, in our culture we tend to focus on the mud that surrounds the diamond. We zoom in on it and try to see what it is made of and examine its elements and properties and spend a lot of time thinking about where the mud came from and what it means that it's on the diamond.

However, have you ever eaten an ice cream cone that's been dipped in chocolate? Sometimes you can take a small bite and a large section of the chocolate coating will shear away. That's what exploring this under-standing is like. As you begin to have insights about your true nature and connect with the wisdom that already exists within you, shifts will begin to happen in ways that don't involve willpower and white knuckles.

The mud that you've been focusing on will begin to shear away, and you'll start to see the diamond that's been there all along.

Your psychological self is part of the wise and wondrous being that knows, among other things, how to heal itself when it receives a physical cut and how to create life from two single cells. There is an infinite, universal intelligence that both guides and powers everything about us, about life on this planet, and about the things beyond our world. This intelligence keeps the stars in the sky; it keeps the earth spinning around the sun. It is in photosynthesis, butterfly migration, and problem-solving crows.

I learned a while back that trees communicate with each other through a network of fungi that grows beneath the earth's surface. With this communication network, the trees can warn each other about threats; they also use it to share water and other resources necessary for survival[1]. How amazing is that? For a long time—millennia—we didn't understand this about trees. But that doesn't mean it wasn't true all that time.

The intelligence that created the trees' ability to communicate is the same intelligence that flows through you at every moment. You could not possibly be separate from it, even if you tried. So, when I say there is nothing wrong with you, this is what I'm pointing toward. You have innocently been focused on the mud that surrounds you and haven't been able to see anything else. Should you choose to continue exploring this understanding, it will become obvious that solutions to any of life's challenges come from looking toward the diamond, not the mud. Eventually, you may even begin to see that the mud was made up by something called thought.

I'm not saying that life doesn't have its challenges. Of course it does. We've all experienced some of those challenges; disappointment, grief, loss, tragedy, abuse, violence and worse. I'm not saying that those things don't happen or that they don't have an effect on us. Of course they do. What I'm pointing toward is that difficult experiences (and happy ones) exist inside the context of your true nature, which is designed as one that is infinitely resilient and innately well. The challenges we experience are drops in the ocean, but they are not the whole ocean.

You are not broken because you cannot be. You may be experiencing a temporary misunderstanding about how your human design works, but that doesn't mean you're broken. You may be misunderstanding the messages from your cravings, but that doesn't mean you're broken. One of the ways I can prove to you that you are infinitely resilient is that you are here, reading this book. I don't know how many times you've failed to curb your cravings, but however many times it was, you picked yourself up and kept going. And here you are, still learning, still trying to resolve that situation.

And I can also prove to you right now that you are made of well-being. The cycle of craving and overeating feels instinctively wrong to you, and not just because our society shames those who overeat. Somewhere inside you, you *know* that there is the potential to feel at peace about food. Even if you've never personally experienced that kind of peace in all your years of searching for it, still, you know it exists. How do you know that? Because you are made of well-being, of peace, and the deepest parts of yourself know that.

# Chapter 7

## *Peristalsis*

I don't know about you, but my experience of trying to tame, control, and conquer my food cravings was like trying to hold a beach ball under water. In a word: exhausting. And in another word: futile. No matter how much force and willpower I applied, no matter how squarely I sat on that ball, the darn thing kept popping up to the surface. My cravings returned, torturing me. So, then I'd try a different way of managing and controlling my overeating habit beach ball, and that wouldn't work either.

What I see now, that I didn't see then, was that I was using the same tool each time to manage the beach ball; it was just wrapped in different packaging.

Diets and weight-loss programs are all the same. They're all trying to teach us new ways of keeping that beach ball submerged. A new program that gets us to count food 'points' instead of calories. A new app that sends us reminders and charts our progress in colorful graphics. A different philosophy about avoiding certain foods and focusing on others. They're all looking at the situation through the same lens: they are all saying that the cravings that lead to overeating are a problem and must be conquered.

The reason diets haven't worked for us up to now is that this premise is flawed.

Don't you think that if conquering cravings was the solution, then we'd have mastered that by now? Don't you think that if human psychology worked that way, then the very first 'diet' or restrictive food program would have provided the answer we were looking for?

What if we're looking at this situation from the wrong angle? What if our cravings are trying to help us, not hurt us? What if learning what they have to say is the thing that resolves them? What might happen if we lean all the way into cravings and try to understand the wisdom they have to offer?

Our culture around the human body does seem to be one of control and domination. Everything from brassieres to running shoes is designed to change and perfect, or at least improve, the way a human body works. It seems to me that this approach works some of the time—I'm sure that anyone who had braces put on to straighten crooked teeth appreciated the end result. But sometimes this 'master and command' approach to our bodies goes a little too far.

Our bodies are innately wise and are *way* more intelligent than we give them credit for when it comes to so many things. Just think about how you came to be: a sperm and an egg collided, and from that moment cells began to divide and divide again. Each time this happens, billions and billions of cells are created with zero input from the mother, other than what her body knows how to do. Eventually the finger cells know that they are finger cells, and the eyeball cells know that they are eyeball cells. How do they know that?! It's beyond our comprehension.

I'm not a doctor, but here are a few more things about our bodies that are mind-bogglingly amazing (but so often go unremarked upon). When you cut yourself, your body knows what to do to heal that cut. When you're cold, your body knows to shiver, which creates heat by contracting and expanding muscles rapidly. Your entire skin-suit renews itself every 28 days. Your liver can regenerate itself. If you wore a pair of goggles called invertoscopes, they would make everything you see appear to be upside down. It would take about 10 days before your brain had adjusted and made everything appear right side up again. You eat things (plant or animal), and your body moves that stuff through roughly 20 feet of intestine, secreting the right enzymes and chemicals at the right times, so that the food is broken down and converted into fuel that keeps you alive. Your body separates what it needs from what it doesn't and gets rid of the latter. You do *nothing* to make any of this happen. Nothing. This happens every day for as long as you are alive.

Come on! Even one of these things knocks my socks off when I think about it. And yet they're all entirely natural and normal.

Let's keep going.

If you break a limb, you receive a message (pain) from your body telling you to not move that limb so that it can heal.

If you move your hand too close to fire, you receive a message from your body telling you to move it away.

If you're about to vomit, you receive messages from your stomach about what's about to happen.

If your shoes are too tight and they're pinching your feet, you loosen the laces.

If you go outside and find that there are drops of water hitting your face, you get an umbrella or put on a rain jacket.

If you're tired you go to sleep.

We trust these signals from our bodies, our feelings, and our senses. We use them to help us navigate through life.

Our food cravings are the same. They are information, feedback from our wise selves. The problems we encounter with failed diets and eating plans occur only because we misunderstand the message. We don't understand the language those cravings are speaking.

And that's why we're here. I'm going to teach you how to speak that language.

# Chapter 8

## *Misunderstanding the Message*

As we discussed in the previous chapter, there are certain messages we receive from our bodies that we're willing to listen to. However, we think of cravings as though they're a broken part of ourselves, like a flat tire on a car or an app on our phone that is on the fritz and keeps sending us unwelcome alerts. What I would like you to consider is that food cravings are actually a barometer. And that barometer is always in perfect working order.

A barometer is a device that tells us about the atmospheric pressure in our geographic area.

A food craving is a feedback system that tells us about the atmospheric pressure within ourselves.

Barometers measure the layers of air that wrap around the earth that are affected by gravity. We call this the earth's atmosphere. Changes in the atmosphere affect the earth's weather systems. The way that a barometer reflects atmospheric pressure is typically with hands (like a clock's hands) on a dial pointing toward numbers.

A food craving is doing exactly the same thing. It is pointing toward the 'weather' inside you.

"Duh," you might say. "If I feel super stressed, I crave a piece of cake. That's not breaking news."

You're right. It's not. But what I'm suggesting is that the craving itself is not an indication that there is anything wrong with you, even when you're feeling stressed or triggered by life. There is wisdom behind the cravings we feel that is deeper than a feeling that we want to use a substance in order to try to soothe and comfort ourselves when we've had a hard day. What I'm saying is that there is a beautiful and perfect mechanism within us (food craving, or any kind of craving) that lets us know what the 'weather' inside us is doing at any given moment. We need that signal (the craving) to remind us of our innate, peaceful nature.

That is the next thing we're going to talk about, and as you'll see, the way it works will have life-changing implications for your overeating habit.

# Chapter 9

## *Meet Nancy*

When you were a child, did you use the expression 'You're not the boss of me'? I did. It was mostly aimed at other kids in the playground or schoolyard, letting them know I wanted to think and act independently.

There is a force, a weather system, within you that can seem as though it's the boss of you, but it isn't. That force is your thinking. Your thoughts.

We tend to move through life obeying our thinking, without even realizing we are doing so. We all have an incessantly chattering, opinionated, sometimes pushy voice within us that tries to run the show—and often succeeds. The voice in our head that sounds like us can be helpful: "I think I'll turn left at this corner," or "Don't bang your face on that open cupboard door." It can be neutral: "I think I'll make some tea," or "My flowers need to be watered." And it can also be critical and judgmental, either about you or others: "Gee, that guy has weird hair," or "Why did I turn left at that corner? That was dumb."

As adults, we live with this running dialogue nearly all the time. It can vary in volume and intensity, but it's nearly always there, like the slightly annoying but also oddly comforting narrator of a nature documentary. Let's call that narrator Nancy. Very often, the comments Narrator Nancy makes are about the circumstances in our lives and whether she approves of them or not. She says things along the lines of, "I should have got that promotion. If I had, my life would be so much better." Or, "The toe fungus I had when I was eight years old is the reason I can't wear running shoes."

Narrator Nancy is very persuasive. We tend to believe what she says, even when she contradicts herself ten minutes later.

What we innocently fail to see is that Nancy is just a part of the documentary that she's narrating. She's not the whole story. She's not the boss, although we sometimes forget this.

Additionally, Nancy can be entirely out of sync with what's going on in front of our faces. You (or I) could be at a lovely event on a beautiful day consisting of the perfect circumstances. (Picture whatever that is for you: a garden, an outdoor musical event, a Civil War battle re-enactment.) The temperature is perfect. You're either surrounded by friends or alone (whichever your preference is). Yet Nancy can be narrating an entirely different experience than this.

"That potato salad that Aunt Jenny served yesterday was atrocious. Why doesn't she ever listen to me about salting the potatoes while they're cooking? It's because my sister Mary has always been her favorite. Jenny has never liked me. It started the moment she saw me with that terrible haircut I got when I was six. That hairdresser was clueless, and Mum wasn't paying attention. Man, I hated those bangs so much. It took me a year to grow them out. Which reminds me, I need to make an appointment for a pedicure soon. Where's my phone?"

Sure, Nancy is often narrating about what's going on in front of us, but just as often she's not. She can go on wild tangents about things that happened years ago. She can also jump to conclusions that aren't based on anything logical, have fierce imaginary arguments with people (the root causes of which are entirely made up), change her point of view on a subject in the blink of an eye, and create fears that turn out to be entirely unfounded. Oh, that Nancy! What a loon. She has moments when she acts like a barrel full of monkeys doing tequila shots.

And yet, we tend to believe she's the boss of us, don't we? We take her at her word about almost anything. Somehow, years ago, without realizing what we were doing, we gave her the keys to the corner office, made her the chairperson of the board, and gave her the unilateral power to make all decisions on our behalf. No wonder she's drunk with power.

However, there is good news. There's a reason Nancy can seem so crazed and yet is also so powerful at times: She is not the boss sitting at the head of the table; she is more like the weather outside your window. Weather that is at times calm, at times violent, and everything in between. A powerful force that is constantly shifting and changing.

Take a look outside right now and make a note of what's happening. For me, it is an extremely pleasant September day as I write this. The sun is shining and it's about 17 degrees Celsius (62.6 degrees Fahrenheit) outside. There's a slight breeze causing the leaves on the trees across the street from me to wave gently. Like I said, extremely pleasant. Fast forward eight hours—or even one hour—from now, though, and we could be in the midst of one of the wild storms that blows in off the Pacific Ocean, bringing with it horizontal rain and wind that buffets and batters everything in its path.

Narrator Nancy, the voice in your head, a.k.a. your thinking, is just like the weather. She is utterly changeable. In fact, change is the main part of her nature.

· · ·

"So what?" you might be thinking. "My moods and thoughts change. Big whoop. What does that have to do with cravings and overeating?"

The answer lies in two surprising, yet woefully neglected, aspects of the human condition:

1. Where the weather moves.

2. Where your experience of that weather comes from.

So, let's talk about these things and why they can help you to peacefully resolve an unwanted overeating habit.

# Chapter 10

## *The Sky*

Some of my favorite memories of my mother are the times when we would have a giggle-fit together. She was the only person who could get me laughing in a way that took my breath away and had tears running down my cheeks. We never knew when these fits would strike or what silly thing would set them off, although it was always a joy when it happened.

I'll give you an example.

One day I was rooting around in the back of the kitchen pantry at my mother and stepfather's house and found that a can of artichoke hearts had burst. There was sticky liquid on the shelf where the can had been, and the mess had also dripped down to the shelves below, so I spent some time cleaning it up. Later, my mum and I were sitting in the living room while my stepfather puttered around in the kitchen.

He must have seen something that prompted him to ask what had happened, so I explained.

When I finished my explanation, he was quiet for a moment and then said, "I don't use artichoke hearts."

Not funny at all, right?

But that little comment set my mum and me off. With one glance at each other, we both burst into hysterical laughing that left us gasping for breath. When this happened, my mum always had a specific way of holding onto her stomach, which I found adorable. We squiggled and squirmed in our chairs while we laughed, and each time the laughter finally started to subside, if we looked at each other it would start up again.

These moments where my mum and I shared a laugh like this are ones I will treasure always. But I tell this family anecdote not for old time's sake but to illustrate a point.

Anytime we had a giggle-fit it would eventually pass, and when that happened, I was always left with the feeling of a storm having passed. You probably know that feeling. It often comes after a big laugh or a big cry. A feeling of being cleansed somehow. In the example I gave you just now, the laughter would fill up my body and soul intensely while it was with me, and then when it moved on I would feel fresh, and also empty, but not in a sad way.

This example points to two primary features of the human condition that are really important to understand when we're learning the language of cravings.

# I. Life works from the inside out.

We live in a world that seems to impact us from the outside in. For example, our spouse leaves their dishes in the sink instead of putting them in the dishwasher and we get angry. We win $50 at bingo and that makes us happy. We see a video on social media about an orphaned armadillo and we feel sad.

However—and this is a big however—what if life actually worked the other way around, from the inside out?

In 1973, a man named Sydney Banks had a profound insight about the way the human experience works. He saw that we actually experience life from the inside out, rather than from the outside in. We don't experience thoughts and feelings as a reaction to what's going on outside of us; rather, we experience thought as an energy flowing through us. He spent the rest of his life sharing this with people because he knew that the impact of understanding this would reduce suffering.

That anger at your spouse about the dishes in the sink isn't about the dishes. It's not even about your spouse. The dishes, and even your spouse's actions, are entirely neutral. The anger you experience is based on your thoughts *about* the dishes and your spouse. "He never does anything I ask," your thoughts say. Or, "Why am I always the one who has to clean up after everyone?" Or, "I don't have time for this today. I'm already late."

When we take the tiniest step back from what we've always believed about how feelings and thoughts work, we begin to understand what Mr. Banks was pointing toward. For example, on one day the dishes in the sink might enrage you. On another day you might not care about them at all. And on a third day you might not even notice them. If our experience really did come from the outside in, you would have the exact same reaction to those dishes every single time. But you don't.

*We live in the world of our thinking,*
*not in the world of our circumstances.*

Our experience of life is *always* coming from within us, based on the thinking we have in that moment.

Here's another way to look at it. If our experience came from the outside in, then everyone who came into your kitchen would feel anger based on the dishes in the sink. But that's not true, is it? Some people might find them amusing. Some might find them sad. Some might not even notice them. The dishes and their location in the sink are entirely neutral.

At any given moment, it is our state of mind that affects what we think about and how we feel about any given situation. If you're in a calm, quiet, content state of mind, those sink-dishes might not faze you. If your thinking is really stirred up and agitated, the sink-dishes might make you feel murderous.

It's important to say that I never, ever expect anyone to swallow what I'm saying whole. This idea is a big one and, speaking personally, it took me some time to get my head around it. So, my recommendation is that you hold it gently as we carry on. We'll come back to it.

## 2. You are the sky.

In the previous chapter we talked about Narrator Nancy and her propensity to try to be the boss of everything, especially you. When we begin to explore the concept that we live in the world of our thinking, it is also possible to see that we are more like a *container* for that thinking than just a robot whose circuitry (thinking) is the only thing driving her behavior.

Here's another mind-blowing concept: You have the ability to observe your own thinking and feeling. It's true that sometimes we get caught up in whatever story Nancy is telling at the moment and, without real-izing it, believe her 100%. But there are other times when we can observe what we're thinking and the resultant feelings we're having. We've all had the experience of being able to reflect on this. "Wow, I was really furious when that blue truck cut me off in traffic today," or "I get so much delight from seeing a cat in a costume." We take these observations for granted, but they're important to notice because what they're telling us is that Nancy isn't the boss of everything (as much as it pains her to hear that).

Descartes famously said, "I think, therefore I am," but that's definitely not the whole story about the human experience. This ability to observe ourselves and reflect on what's going on with us, sometimes even while it's going on, is the larger part of who we are. Even when we're blind to this.

You are the dwelling where Nancy lives. She is a tenant in that house, not the house itself. To add a new metaphor to the mix, your thoughts and feelings are like the weather, and you are the sky that the weather moves through. Our ability to observe that weather tells us that we are not the weather. If we were *just* the weather, and nothing else, we wouldn't be able to do that. If Nancy really was the boss, we wouldn't be able to observe her antics.

Taking this metaphor further, the sky cannot be affected by the weather. It is always there, no matter how dark the clouds are or how many storms are passing through. The sky is entirely unaffected by the weather. Have you ever seen a damaged sky? Has the sky ever been torn or broken or even scratched by the tornadoes and hurricanes and lightning that passes through it?

No, of course not.

Knowing that our thoughts and feelings are not the entirety of who we are, that these are things that move *through* us, is another one of the keys to understanding the secret language of cravings. When we see Nancy for who she is and begin to understand that she is not the whole story of who we are, that leads to a new awareness of the real purpose our food cravings serve. We'll talk about that in the next chapter.

In the meantime, my gentle suggestion is that you take the two ideas from this chapter away with you and, for the next few hours or days, see if you can see any examples of them at work in your life.

Be the observer and see if you notice how your state of mind affects your thinking and your emotions in various situations.

Are you able to see the natural way your thoughts and feelings move? You may notice that they are a bit like a river: constantly in motion, flowing and changing moment to moment.

# Chapter 11

## *Insight and Wisdom*

S o, if we pay less attention to Nancy and her incessant chatter, what *should* we be listening to?

I'm fairly certain you are up to your eyeballs in knowledge about calorie counts, energy expended, and carbohydrates. Those of us who have been fighting an overeating battle for years could have PhDs in these subjects. Yet, how much change has all that knowledge created? In my case, it was zero. After 30 years of learning everything I could about my overeating habit, I felt like I could have taught classes on any one of the strategies I'd tried. It was pretty frustrating to know so much while also being on the receiving end of F grades in everything I tried.

It turns out that what I needed wasn't knowledge; it was insight and wisdom.

Insight and wisdom are the twins that help bring about change. They are, always have been, and always will be within you. There is nothing you need to do or be or have in order to access them.

Competing for our attention are knowledge and understanding, which are the noisier, more attention-getting pair. Insight and wisdom are subtler and quieter, but also more profound. Lasting change comes about because of insight and wisdom.

We are hard wired for insight, just as we are hard wired for peace and well-being. We all have insights all the time about all kinds of things in life. Speaking personally, it wasn't until I began exploring this under-standing that I learned that insight is something I can rely on to help me at any given moment, with any situation.

Our minds are problem-solving machines, and for that we are grateful. But they are also like the artificial intelligence (AI) that's been in the news so much lately; they only know what they know. So, in the same way that AI is fed with information that was already in existence, our minds, our thinking, prefer to look for answers in what they already know. Our minds are like a closed-loop system. You've probably had an experi-ence of this: you've got a particularly perplexing problem that doesn't have an obvious or appealing answer, so your mind just keeps looping around to the three or four solutions it can come up with. Inside

your head, this might sound like, "If I do X
be unhappy about Y. But if I do A or B then [ano
problem] will crop up." I've had times where I've
stayed trapped in a loop like that for days, like a leaf
caught in a whirlpool.

There is an alternative to this approach, thankfully,
and when I began learning to rely on it, my life felt so
much more peaceful and safe. That alternative is
simply this: relying on the insights we all receive from
the intelligence of the universe that surrounds us, and
of which we are all an integral part. We've touched on
this universal intelligence earlier in the book, when we
talked about cravings actually being a part of that
intelligence. And here it is, cropping up again.

Let's do a little visual exercise:

1. Picture a large container. It can be as large as you
want it to be—the size of a travel trunk or a ship-
ping container or Windsor Castle—just as long as it's
a container that is closed on all of its sides. Now
imagine that within that container is all the knowledge your mind has: everything it knows about
things like gardening and putting Ikea furniture
together and long division and raising children and
training dogs and plot lines from *Friends* and options
for meals this evening and how to get to the movie
theater and mortgage rates and how to use a shovel
and facts about starfish and constellations and geese
migration. Your mind really does know a *lot* of stuff.
All this knowledge is inside that container you

go. Everything fits in there very

the Pacific Ocean. It's so big, of
won't be able to picture all of it, but
of it as you can; the wide open, blue-
green waves ... h whitecaps stretching so far away that
there's no land in sight in any direction you look.

3. Finally, picture the container you filled with all your mind's knowledge floating in the middle of that huge body of water. No matter how large your container, compared to the ocean it is like a wine cork floating almost invisibly on that vast, depthless expanse.

That ocean you pictured represents the universal intelligence and infinite possibilities that are available to us at all times, including when we encounter a problem. We are, at every moment, swimming in a sea of intelligence. Our minds like to think they know it all and can answer every question, and they do answer lots of questions brilliantly, but as I mentioned a moment ago, our minds are really a closed-loop system. They know what they know. And often the answers to our challenges lie outside what we already know.

The really exciting thing about this universal intelligence is that it's always there for us, even when we're unaware of it. There's nothing you need to do to access it or to become worthy of it. You are part of it, the same way you are part of the oxygen you breathe.

Real, lasting change comes about because of insights we experience that originate in this sea of universal intelligence. When we suddenly see a situation or a problem in a new way, we can never un-see it. It's that moment when you've been pushing on a door to get into a building and it won't budge—and then you realize you have to pull to get it to open.

Albert Einstein said, "I believe in intuition and inspiration... At times I feel certain I am right while not knowing the reason." What I'm describing as insight, Einstein described as intuition and inspiration. It's all the same thing. A light bulb moment. Oprah Winfrey calls these 'Ah-ha moments.' Suddenly, you see things differently, and even though nothing has changed, everything is different.

As I said, we all know a tremendous amount about calories in/calories out, carbohydrates, and avoiding sugar. There's a lot of information in our brains about these things. Yet, all that understanding hasn't changed a thing; otherwise, you wouldn't be here.

Remember when we talked about how managing an overeating habit is like trying to keep a beach ball submerged under the water? Insight is the thing that deflates that beach ball. With each insight you have about your innate well-being, how your human design really works, and this paradigm of health we're exploring together, that beach ball that you've been trying to manage for so long will lose some of its air.

Eventually, you'll notice the ball isn't even there any longer; there will be nothing left for you to manage. When we explore this inside-out understanding, of course we're learning things and taking in information. And we're also having insights about our human design.

Have you ever read *Eat, Pray, Love* by Elizabeth Gilbert? In the beginning of that book, Gilbert explains the circumstances that were about to springboard her into taking a journey around the world to Italy, India, and Indonesia. She had been suffering. She had a life that she felt should have been making her happy: a husband, a nice house in the Hudson Valley as well as an apartment in Manhattan, couple friends, parties and picnics, and weekends spent in big box stores buying appliances. But it was a life that wasn't fitting her properly. And, crucially, her husband wanted children and she was beginning to realize that maybe she didn't. But she felt terrible because she thought she should want them.

So, we find her lying on her bathroom floor in the middle of a cold November night, sobbing and praying. She's looking for answers about what to do in her marriage and in her life. She wants Big Answers to her Big Questions. She wants God to tell her what to do with her marriage, with her womb, and with her life. And she does get an answer, although it's not the one she expects. Within her, a voice comes, and it says, "Go back to bed, Liz."[1]

In the book, she states that she knew this was wisdom because "[t]rue wisdom gives the only possible answer at any given moment and that night going back to bed was the only possible answer."[2] She goes on to explain that in hindsight she saw that she didn't need to know all the Big Answers to her life's Big Questions in the middle of the night on a cold bathroom floor. What she needed was to take the next small step and take care of herself. In that moment this translated to going back to bed. She needed rest, not a grand pronouncement about what to do with the rest of her life. She also describes experiencing feelings of warm affection from the voice and that it sounded like her own voice, "but perfectly wise, calm and compassionate."[3]

I love this example, because it illustrates so vividly our inner knowing, our wisdom and insight, and how they communicate with us. One of the things I resonate with in this story is the feeling Liz experienced when she heard that message: "perfectly wise, calm and compassionate." This is the alternative to Nancy.

Elizabeth Gilbert heard this voice in a pretty dramatic way at a time that must have felt like a scary crossroads for her. But we don't need to travel to the depths of despair to be able to connect with the wise, calm, compassionate aspect of ourselves. It is there, always, no matter what.

I understand if you're tempted to dismiss this concept as a lot of new age nonsense. Culturally, especially in North America, we are not taught the value of or even the presence of our connection to our innate, compassionate wisdom. We are largely a left-brained society and, as previously discussed, can be very attached to what our minds already know. But I wonder if you've ever had an experience of connecting with your own wisdom. It might have been a very small, quiet moment where you just *knew* something. It may have been so quiet that you dismissed it, only later realizing with hindsight that something had spoken the truth to you.

We can never turn Nancy off; it is her job to be with us, chattering, all the time. She is the weather flowing through the sky. Life wouldn't be the same without her. But the reason I bring this up is that accessing your innate wisdom is the alternative to only ever listening to Nancy. We can spend our lives caught up in all of Nancy's drama without realizing there's an alternative to her often-fearful narrative. And we are never separate from that which wishes to speak to us calmly, quietly, wisely. Wisdom is always there. We don't have to do anything to conjure it. It is like the air we breathe: always there for us but so often unnoticed.

Nancy can be harsh and critical. She can be neutral while being smart, but she can also be bossy.

Wisdom never comes with any of this sort of energy and attitude.

Nancy is all rules and regulations and drawing inside the lines.

Wisdom is love.

Nancy likes to tell us what to do and why it matters and how what she's saying makes perfect sense. (Until she changes her mind, at which point she'll tell us why *that* makes sense.)

Wisdom has a really good feeling to it. You know for sure you can trust it. There's no fanfare; it just feels *right*.

Nancy is a parade with marching bands, colorful floats, and acrobats.

Wisdom is a leopard in the bush; strong, nearly silent, powerful.

Nancy likes to think she's the boss (and acts like it).

Wisdom is never, ever bossy. Wisdom is *knowing*.

Nancy can be fearful and anxious.

Wisdom is always calm. Never fearful or anxious.

While no one, perhaps with the exception of Winnie-the-Pooh, hears wisdom and insight speak to them at every moment of their lives, we can learn to listen for their presence, and we can learn to rely on them. Nancy will never stop chatting, but we can learn that it is possible to turn to another, wiser source to help us make decisions. Coming to understand that wisdom and insight are always available to us means that we are less likely to be blown around by Nancy's moods.

But what does this have to do with resolving an overeating habit? Well, it's an important part of the larger picture of who you are. There is so much more to you than the content of Nancy's storms. When we explore this and experience it for ourselves, wisdom and insight become a safe place from which to navigate our lives, bringing us what we need in order to see our unwanted habit for what it really is.

# Chapter 12

## *Your Innate Mental Health*

Your overeating habit is a sign of your mental health.

Yes, really.

We touched on this in an earlier chapter, and I want to explore it more deeply now.

When we have an unwanted habit like overeating it can feel like there's something broken about us. Our culture tends to shame those who overeat, and it is widely assumed that there is something wrong with anyone who has an overeating habit. Both we and others make judgments about the lack of discipline that we seem to be exhibiting when we overeat; we may hear that overeating signals that we are incapable of self-care, or that we lack even a basic understanding of calories and nutritional requirements. You've heard it all. I know I have.

But what if an unwanted habit like overeating was a sign of all that's *right* with you, not with something that's wrong?

What if it is a solution, not a problem?

Pop quiz: What do Cruella de Vil, the 2015 Chicago Cubs, and Taylor Swift have in common?

Answer: They all want something.

Cruella wants Dalmatian puppies so that she can make a fancy fur coat (yikes!). For 108 years the Cubs wanted (and failed) to win the World Series of baseball. And Ms. Swift seems to want to entertain the world.

You have something in common with all of these folks: you want something, probably several somethings. Maybe not the World Series, but perhaps a different home or a new car or tickets to a sold-out Taylor Swift show.

We all want things. It's part of the human condition. Right now, my wants include having the pain in my arthritic index finger go away, writing something today that will help people, and finding a fabric I like for a chair I want to have reupholstered.

Very often, though, what we want isn't as much about the object of our affection as it is about how we think we'll feel when we get that thing. A Rolls Royce is an inanimate object and doesn't actually have the ability to make someone feel important, but we can mistakenly believe it does. My brother used to wear a style of sunglasses that I thought were somewhat goofy-looking until I realized he chose that style because it's what baseball players wear. (He was a huge baseball fan.) The glasses, he believed, made him look cool like his favorite baseball players. I carry a purse from a brand that a British princess uses because my thinking tells me it makes me more…princessy.

If we drill down a little further and get existential about our wants, what we'll see is that so often what we're looking for is a different, better feeling. We're almost always trying to feel better. I've used examples above of material things that we use when we're searching for a better feeling, but just about anything we do is motivated by the same quest. Here are some examples I've thought of as I've been exploring this:

- a university student snuggles down on the couch for a night with a favorite movie
- a husband lashes out at his spouse about something inconsequential
- a bully picks on someone
- a woman buys herself a new set of makeup brushes, even though she has six unused sets at home
- a driver honks and curses at someone who cut her off in traffic

- a chef makes a delicious meal for friends
- a woman who feels she is 20 pounds overweight eats three donuts for breakfast

Each of these things (and trillions of others) are examples of how we search for a better feeling. Some might be obvious, like the women buying or eating something unnecessary, or the student watching a movie. But the other examples are motivated by the same desire.

Let's look at the example of the bully. That person is also trying to feel better, to find a better feeling. A number of things are probably going on for that person. It is likely that they are being bullied themselves or grew up being bullied. As a result, the thinking they're experiencing about themselves is painful; it is probably habitually harsh and negative. So, when the bully bullies someone else they get some temporary relief from the painful thoughts they have. They are momentarily distracted from their suffering while their attention is focused on someone else.

In other words, to the bully the bullying behavior feels like a solution. It momentarily helps the bully to feel slightly better. It provides relief from the storm of painful thinking the bully spends most of their life in.

Whether we're reaching for something that looks like it is comforting (shopping, eating, alcohol) or engaging in a behavior that looks destructive or mean, the motivation is the same: we're always searching for a better feeling.

Do you own an Instant Pot? They were all the rage a few years ago. (I love mine.) Instant Pots are a brand name of what my grandmother called a pressure cooker, which is a pot that cooks its contents with pressure in addition to heat. The pot is sealed and pressure builds up, and that's what cooks whatever's inside, far more quickly than with just heat itself.

Here's a metaphor for this most natural of human phenomena: our heads are like pressure cookers, and our behavior is the release valve on that pressure cooker.

If you own either an Instant Pot or a pressure cooker you know that there's a valve that allows you to release some of the pressure in the pot. When you do so, it makes a whooshing sound, and you can see steam escaping the pot.

The thinking you experience in life is like the contents of that pressure cooker. It can build and build until it feels like too much to cope with, swirling around inside your noggin, keeping you awake at night, interfering with the concentration required for other things. The solution for the build-up of this pressure is the release valve. Behaviors like the ones I listed above are all a sort of release valve—lashing out, over-shopping, yelling in traffic, overeating, bullying someone.

The release valve gets us back to a better feeling. Even if the change is only incremental we still feel a bit better. Some of the pressure within us has been released and we are slightly more calm, more peaceful. This is what I'm referring to when I say that an overeating habit is a *solution*, not a problem. That habit is releasing some of the pressure within you. It is a necessary and natural part of your perfect design. Without the release valve, the pressure cooker would explode. Without your overeating habit, you would, well, maybe not explode, but you'd definitely be more uncomfortable.

This is how your habit is a sign of your mental health. That release valve behavior is evidence that you are looking for a better feeling, that you are wired to crave and search for a good feeling. What that tells us is that you are made of peace and well-being, and your habit is evidence of that. Just like a fish will always need water, humans will always need what they are made of: peace, love, well-being. Your habit is a truth about who you are at your core.

When you experience a craving, that feeling is letting you know that there is too much pressure in your Instant Pot.

So, what's the alternative? We all live with thoughts in our heads, so how can we release the "thought pressure" that builds up without turning toward our unwanted overeating habit? Well, here's where things get really interesting. Unlike other self-help tools, I'm not going to direct you toward replacing the pressure value release with some other sort of behavior. Instead, using a different metaphor, we're going to look at the nature of what's in the pot itself.

# Chapter 13

## *Bathtubs*

At this point in our exploration, you might be thinking that what I'm talking about in this book is positive thinking, or changing our thoughts so that they are working for us instead of against us. Changing our thoughts so that they don't build up in the pressure cooker.

But that's not what this is.

In order to explain, let me switch metaphors from the one in the previous chapter. Imagine you lived in a world where no one had explained to you how a bathtub drain works. Every time you took a bath, afterwards you'd have to find a way to empty the water out of the tub. You might take a bucket and scoop out the water and carry it through your house to the front door, and then take it outside and dump it somewhere. Then you'd have to go back to the tub and scoop out some more water and carry that outside, repeating that process until all the water was out of the tub. Emptying the tub would require a lot of effort on your part and create a lot of extra stress for you. Plus, there would be mess to clean up afterward in the form of drips and puddles of water on the floor of your home.

Not knowing any other way to empty a tub, you'd go through this laborious process every time you took a bath until the day someone explained to you how drains work. They'd show you that there is a drain on the bottom of the tub that, when open, allows the water to flow away on its own. They'd demonstrate that there was nothing else for you to do except open that drain. Once you saw this, you'd never empty the tub with a bucket again.

The understanding that I'm exploring in this book is like that information about the drain. I'm pointing out to you how tubs, drains, and water work. If it's not clear, the water represents your thinking. As you begin to understand this, and as your understanding deepens, you'll see there's less and less for you to do with your thinking.

Our thinking flows into us from a source other than ourselves; Sydney Banks called this source Mind. It stays with us for a time, and then moves on without us having to do anything about it. Sometimes the water is crystal clear, sometimes it is murky, but the thing that never changes is that it flows, it moves of its own accord. That is its nature.

Continuing with the metaphor, if we took a 'positive thinking' approach, we would be trying to control the clarity of the water that comes into the tub. That's a ton of work, and it's fruitless because the nature of water is that some days it's clear, and some days it's not. (Where I live, when we have big rainstorms the water can get very murky indeed.) Being concerned with the quality of the water in the tub at any given moment (positive thinking) is a waste of energy because in the next moment there will be different water in the tub. And then again in the moment after that.

Instead, when we focus on understanding the nature of water, knowing it will continue to flow no matter what, we can relax about what the tub is holding at any given moment.

Our behaviors like overeating are always an accurate reflection of the quality of the thinking we're experiencing. For example, the bully we met earlier is simply experiencing a perpetually low quality of thinking. In the case of overeating, when we don't understand this dynamic, we try to force our behaviors to change with things like diets. Each new kind of diet looks like a solution, but really, they're all just new and better-marketed ways for moving the water from the tub with the bucket.

Resolving an overeating habit doesn't come from forcing behavioral change; it comes from understanding the nature of thought.

# Chapter 14

## *The Dog Has to Pee*

Here's the one simple reason all the strategies and tactics I mentioned in the chapter where I introduced myself don't help us to resolve an overeating habit: they ask us to look in the wrong direction.

Have you ever been to London, England? I first visited that historic city in 1997 as a very naive but energetic 29-year-old. One of the things I noticed almost immediately was that painted on the roads, especially at crosswalks, was the instruction to 'Look Right.' It took me a moment to understand why this was: when I was about to cross the road, I automatically looked left for oncoming cars. I come from a country where the vehicles drive on the right side of the road, so they approach from my left when I'm at a crosswalk. However, in the UK the vehicles drive on the left, so looking left at a crosswalk before you step onto the road just means you won't see the king's Bentley as it mows you down.

All the strategies and tactics we've tried to tame our cravings and our overeating habit have had us looking in the wrong direction. They ask us to look in the direction of the *behaviors* that our cravings create and then to manage, correct, or control those. However, the solution actually lies in the other direction, looking at *why* the craving exists in the first place. In this analogy, behaviors are 'downstream,' while the root cause of craving is 'upstream.'

Let's use an example to illustrate this. There's a dog that's been scratching at the inside of a front door. It has damaged the paint and the finishing on the door and the frame. So, the dog's owner tries to manage and correct that behavior: she tries to bribe the dog with treats to come away from the door. She installs padding on the lower parts of the door to protect the paint. She tries to lock the dog out of the room where the front door is. She uses a shock collar, and every time the dog scratches at the door it receives a mild electrical shock intended to curb the behavior. You get the idea.

All of these strategies and tactics, while logical and well-intentioned, are downstream from the real problem. Upstream, the real problem is simply that *the dog has to pee*. Let the dog out into the yard and the problem is solved.

Our cravings are like that dog. They're desperately trying to tell us something, and we keep telling them to sit down and be quiet. We muzzle the messages our cravings are sending us by using diets and food plans.

When cravings are speaking to us, they want us look upstream at their origin. The dog in our example speaks with its body and its actions because it has no words. In the same way, our internal, innate wisdom speaks with our feelings.

I'm going to repeat that so you don't miss it: Our internal, innate wisdom speaks with our feelings.

When we look upstream, we see that our cravings are letting us know that we're caught up in our thinking. If no one has taught us the flowing nature of thought or that we are the sky that our thinking moves through, then we innocently take every storm very seriously. We're living life at 120 km/h when we could be cruising along sedately like a raft on a gentle river. We're innocently attached to our busy, insecure thoughts because we're unaware of the ocean of wisdom we live in.

Downstream from this are the behaviors that show up to let us know the state of our thinking: things like eating an entire bag of cookies while watching TV in the evening or devouring potato chips and cheese puffs every day at lunch.

If you go to alexandraamor.com/secretresources you'll find a printable chart I've created that compares what we see when we look downstream versus upstream. You can also listen to Q&A episode 22 of my podcast Unbroken about this subject.

I used to think that the specifics of my overeating habit were what I should learn more about in order to correct my behavior. For example, I often wrestled with over-snacking in the evening, finding myself going back to the kitchen cupboards looking for bags of salt and vinegar potato chips, or crackers and cheese. I wasn't hungry, but I felt deep cravings for salty, crunchy snacks. Given my familiarity with the old, pathology-based paradigm of psychology, I would examine what it could be about the time of day between supper and bed that was creating cravings in me. I overturned every rock in my psyche looking for past experiences of trauma or even just discontent that might have happened at that time of day, anything at all that could be linked to my snacky behavior in the present. Maybe it was because my dad and his second wife, both emotionally abusive alcoholics, were home at that time of day, creating chaos and making me feel unsafe. Maybe I had traumatic memories of being lonely and scared at that time of day.

We are taught to look to the past for clues about what's happening in the present. Our cultural psychological zeitgeist also points us in this direction, so it makes sense that this was where I looked to try to end my snacking habit. The only problem with that strategy was that it didn't work. No matter how much talk therapy I had about my upbringing, no matter how many emotionally draining journaling exercises I did, no matter how many sad/bad/scary memories I tried to remember in order to resolve them, I continued to overeat in the evening, as well as other times of day.

I was looking in the wrong direction. Innocently. I didn't know there was an alternative to the approach I was taking. I thought it was the only option. And I thought it hadn't worked because I hadn't turned over enough rocks. So, I kept looking, kept searching for more crappy memories like they were emotional boils that needed to be lanced. I kept looking downstream, hoping that once I'd found them all, I'd be free.

What I really needed was to look in an entirely different direction. I needed to look upstream, toward my innate health, and understand that my cravings were not telling me that something about me was broken: they were telling me that I was working perfectly. They were saying, "Hey, your natural state of being is one of calm and peace and connection with universal wisdom. When you forget that, we'll let you know. We'll remind you with a feeling that's uncomfortable so that you pay attention."

# Chapter 15

## *What Cravings Are Really Saying*

Cravings let us know the state of our thinking.

It's that simple.

I'm not a parent, so I've never had the experience of raising children. For this reason, perhaps, I admire it when I'm in a public place and I see a parent handling a child's meltdown in a skillful and compassionate way. What I see in these instances is that the parents don't take the meltdown personally. They gently hold the space for the child to express her feelings, while at the same time not being indulgent or—perhaps more importantly—reacting to the meltdown. They seem to know that the meltdown will blow through, like a storm, and when it's done it will move on.

Looking back at our discussion about Narrator Nancy, when we are taking her meltdowns and tantrums really seriously it is our cravings that let us know we're doing that. Our feelings (for example, cravings, but also discomfort, urgency, anxiety, etc.) are always letting us know how much we're caught up in our thinking. That is, how seriously we're taking Nancy. Remember a few chapters back when we talked about cravings being a barometer? This is how they do that.

It works like this:

Part 1. Our thinking (Nancy) is really stirred up from, for example, a rough day at work or a fight with a friend. Or it could just be habitually stirred up and insecure.

Part 2. We feel a craving. "Man! I need several glasses of wine, half a chocolate cake, and a family-sized bag of potato chips."

Part 3. We respond to the craving by eating something because we know from experience this works to make us feel better. (More on this in a minute.)

Now, here's a really important point that I want you to make special note of: in part 3 of the scenario above, you are taking care of yourself. Remember that having that wine/cake/potato chips is a solution, not a problem. You are not sabotaging yourself, as so many diet gurus try to convince us. You are not self-harming or deliberately being mean to yourself. You are not an addict.

Hear this: *You are doing what makes sense in the moment.*

As I said, it works! Giving in to our cravings works. It settles our thinking down. It calms us. It distracts us from the (temporary) storm of feelings and thoughts inside us. In other words, responding to a craving shuts Nancy up for a little while; therefore, doing this is a sign of our mental health.

Alternatively, here's what this same scenario looks like when we understand the language of cravings:

Part 1. Our thinking (Nancy) is really stirred up from, for example, a rough day at work or a fight with a friend. Or it could just be habitually stirred up and insecure.

Part 2. We feel a craving. "Man! I need several glasses of wine, half a chocolate cake, and a family-sized bag of potato chips."

Part 3. We notice that feeling of craving and remember that it is a signal from our innate wisdom that our thinking is really stirred up. And we know that there's nothing we need to do to get that thinking to change. It will settle down on its own because we are designed that way. It is a storm that will move on, just like a toddler's tantrum.

In the past, because we innocently misunderstood the message from our cravings, we got all tangled up in how to suppress the cravings, conquer the cravings, ignore the cravings, which entirely misses the point.

Which is why diets don't work. They're focused on entirely the wrong thing.

The reason our cravings return again and again (in my case for 30 years) is that we've misunderstood the message they're trying to deliver. We think they're an indication that we're broken or flawed, that we're unable to deal with stress, when actually what they're pointing out is that we work perfectly. They are pointing out that our *thinking* is really stirred up and that this is not a good time to make decisions or to even trust what Nancy is saying. They are reminding us that our natural state of being is one of peace, well-being, and calm.

The good news is that because our thoughts and feelings are moving through us, like the water moves through the bathtub and the weather moves through the sky, we can rest easy knowing that we will always return to our natural state of peace and calm. As Maya Angelou says, "Every storm runs out of rain." The blue sky always returns, no matter how long the storm lasts.

The more we notice this, and the more we have insights about our true nature, the less our cravings will need to get our attention. They will drop away on their own because they are no longer needed.

# Chapter 16

## *The Call Toward Home*

For decades I believed that what my food cravings were pointing toward or alerting me to was brokenness within me. I innocently thought that cravings were pointing toward things like unresolved childhood traumas or emotional injuries from the past. I thought they were pointing toward 'issues' I needed to resolve.

We believe this because that's what our most well-understood psychological paradigm tells us.

Perhaps, like me, you've spent years or decades trying to resolve those issues so that your cravings would go away. We innocently believe a) that we can be wounded, b) that those wounds will continue to torment us for as long as we're alive, and c) that we can then use substances like food to comfort ourselves from that torment.

Alexandra Amor

But what if we misunderstand the way that events from the past affect us? What if that old psychological paradigm is pointing us in the wrong direction? What if *that's* why none of the strategies and tactics we've tried in order to stop overeating have worked? It's not that we were doing it wrong or were beyond repair, it's that we misunderstood the assignment, as the kids these days say.

We sometimes think that food cravings are alerting us to wounds from the past and problems within our psychological or emotional being that need to be healed. In fact, cravings are trying to point out to us that we were never wounded in the first place. They are calling us home to our true nature, to the fact that we are infinitely resourceful, resilient, and whole. They are letting us know that we are in a temporary misunderstanding about how our thinking works.

Our experience of life comes not from life itself, but from how we think about it.

Now, please understand, I'm *not* saying that your traumas and wounds and experiences in the past don't exist or that they don't matter. Not at all. These things have contributed toward making us who we are, just as our happy, fulfilling experiences have. What I am saying is that looking in the direction of our innate resilience and the well-being that exists within us is what resolves unwanted habits. Seeing the true nature of thought is what brings peace.

Dr. Bill Pettit, who was board-certified in adult, adolescent, and geriatric psychiatry, and in psychosomatic (mind-body) medicine, learned about the ideas that I'm sharing in this book from the man who first articulated them, Sydney Banks. The logo on Dr. Pettit's website is a cork floating in water, which symbolizes that our human design is one that, without effort and without interference from our minds, will always return to its natural state of rested well-being. We don't need help getting to a calm, quiet state; we naturally go there, even when we're stressed out or unhappy.

We've all experienced moments of this: a hearty laugh in the midst of a deep depression; a few moments during a very stressful period where our mind falls quiet, and we lose track of time; a peaceful feeling amid chaos; a loving or compassionate feeling toward someone who is 'difficult.' These experiences, momentary though they might be, point us toward the true nature of our design.

But what about illness, you might ask. What about disease and physical and mental challenges? How can I say that we are well and whole when we experience things like cancer and epilepsy?

Let's use an example to illustrate what I'm pointing toward. Have you ever been in a bad mood? If so, did that mood encompass all of who you are? Would you define yourself by that mood?

Or was it temporary? Did it exist in the context of your larger personality? Was it something that you experienced but not all of who you are?

Without trying to be too reductive, that bad mood is an illustration of what all of our life experiences are like, whether they are insignificant or enormous. They exist in the greater context of who we are, which is spiritual beings having a human experience. Even when we are gravely ill, we are part of something greater than just the momentary human experience we are having. There is something more to us than our skin and bones and arthritic knees. There is a part of us that is always well and whole.

Your food cravings are calling you home to that 'something more.' They are a part of the same universal intelligence that brings the blossoming trees to life in the spring and guides the gray whales from Alaska to Hawaii and back again. They are asking you to stop and reflect about who you really are. Are you an amalgamation of all your thoughts and experiences? Or do those things exist within the context of something greater?

Remember, this is not dogma. I promise I'm not trying to sell you a religion. What is resonating with you about what I'm saying (if anything)? That's the place to explore.

# Chapter 17

## *Snow Globe*

I've been a little disparaging about Narrator Nancy, and I need to make amends about that, because she too is part of our perfect, and perfectly kind, human design. All it takes for Nancy to have less of a grip on us is seeing her for who she is and how she works. She's actually a gift, and a creative gift at that. Where would we be without the gift of thought?

One of the most interesting characteristics of Nancy's —that is, your—thinking is that it's a bit like the flecks in a snow globe. You know the type of glass globes I mean; they're filled with a watery fluid and have a scene inside—the New York City skyline or the Eiffel Tower. And they also have a carpet of small flakes that, when the snow globe is still, look like snow resting on the ground. When you shake the snow globe the flakes fly around, simulating a snowstorm. When you set the snow globe down, the flakes settle, eventually all coming to rest on the floor of the globe again.

Our thinking and our psychological state are exactly like that snow globe. When we leave them alone, they settle down on their own. Set the globe down and do nothing else and the little storm of flakes will stop swirling. Our minds' default way of being is one of calm and quiet. That's when we are present—to ourselves, to our loved ones and friends, to nature, to life. It's also when we are more receptive to the wisdom and insight that are always available to us from the infinitely intelligent universe.

Unfortunately, when we don't know this, what we tend to do with problems or challenges like food cravings is add more thinking to the mix. We continue shaking up the snow globe—adding more thinking to a problem or concern—because we don't know we have the ability to set it down. Adding more thinking to a problem isn't helpful, and yet we continue to do it because we don't know there's an alternative.

Have you ever been in a difficult or upsetting situation where you needed to make a decision or a choice but found yourself stymied? Maybe your mind was busy leaping from one potential answer to another, unable to settle or to convince you that any of the answers it was coming up with were right. That's the snow globe effect.

Building on this, have you ever mentally walked away from a situation like that and found that the answer to the problem popped into your head when you weren't thinking about it? Maybe you decided to take a nap or watch pimple popping videos on YouTube. Maybe you went for a walk or distracted yourself with a pleasurable activity. Then, suddenly, the answer comes to you from out of nowhere. And you know it's right. The answer has a quality of peace and rightness about it, and it's probably not something you had thought of earlier in your stirred-up state. It's an 'outside the box' answer.

This is what happens when we set the swirling snow globe down. When we stop shaking it up with more and more thinking, and instead let the storm settle so that our innate wisdom can get through to us, insightful answers are often the result.

I'll give you a personal example: in 2017 I had temporarily moved from British Columbia to Ontario and was living with my mother and stepfather. Prior to this I had lived in a large city for about 30 years. For almost the entire time I had lived in that city, I had yearned to move to a small town where I could walk to everything, spend time in nature, and write. Circumstances hadn't allowed that, but it had not stopped being a dream of mine.

Unfortunately, shortly after I arrived in Ontario my mother began receiving hospice care and I knew my time in her town would soon be coming to an end. I began to consider where I would go after my mother's passing. I was a bit troubled about this and about how I would make the right choice for the next stage in my life. It seemed like a big deal and the weight of that made me a little anxious. In addition to the grief I was feeling about losing my mum, I could feel myself stewing about this decision I needed to make. So, one day I sat down with my journal and was preparing to organize my thoughts by writing down the locations I'd considered moving to in the past and maybe make some 'pros and cons' lists to help me with my decision. However, as I opened my journal and poised my pen over the blank page, a knowing came over me. "It's Ucluelet," the feeling said. "It's always been Ucluelet."

Somehow, in that moment, I knew in my bones that this was the right choice about where to live. Not only did the realization come with a knowing about its rightness, but I also felt like this knowing had been there all along, just waiting for me to notice it. Interestingly, if I had got around to making my pro-and-con lists, I doubt that Ucluelet would even have made it into the top ten places I was considering moving to. But thankfully, before I could get too caught up in my thinking about the decision I had to make, wisdom stepped in and gave me the answer. I've been in Ucluelet ever since and hope to never have to leave.

I also experience this in my creative life nearly every day. When I'm doing creative work like writing or creating online courses, I'll sometimes be wrestling with how to clearly express an idea or find an interesting way to tell a story. If the wrestling goes on too long, I know I need a break. When I get up from my chair to get some water or go to the bathroom, I set the problem, and my thinking about it, down for just a moment or two, and more often than not suddenly the solution to whatever I was wrestling with pops into my head. Walks are also great for this. While I'm noticing the trees and the good smells from the rainforest, and my mind is both distracted and settled, insight and wisdom can step in. I have learned not to walk without my phone because it is what I use to record the ideas I have while I'm walking.

The secrets that the language of cravings is trying to share with us are not found within the storms of thinking that we experience. Adding more thinking to the 'problem' of an overeating habit (or any problem) is not going to solve it. Thinking that involves self-blame, shame, and self-judgment about overeating only shakes up the snow globe. So does searching for new strategies and tactics to manage our cravings. When we're in the middle of a whirling, ferocious snowstorm we can't hear the wisdom within us, and within our cravings. Thankfully, we simply need to make a new habit of noticing that our thinking storms settle down on their own, without any interference from us. And when they do, the innate wisdom that lives within all of us can speak.

The next time you encounter a problem or challenge in your life, try experimenting with it. Try metaphorically setting the problem down. Set it aside mentally, let yourself and your thinking settle, and then just wait. See what happens and/or what occurs to you from that settled place. You might find that either the problem resolves itself, or you experience an insight about how to resolve it.

## Chapter 18

### *Why Diets Work Temporarily*

But wait, you might say. Why do diets sometimes work temporarily?

I've had the experience, and perhaps you have as well, where for the first two or three days, maybe a week at the outside, a new eating plan that I was on really seemed to work. It would feel easy, and I would be energized and excited about it. And then the wheels would fall off. For me, the longest I could ever last on a new diet was maybe a week. This happened over and over and over again.

As I began to explore the inside-out understanding I looked at the question of why diets work temporarily, and what I saw was that the occasional, temporary success of a diet or new eating plan actually proved what this understanding is pointing toward.

When we have an overeating habit, we suffer. We don't want to be overweight; we also don't want to have the habit itself, and the habit can have a really detrimental effect on our lives. Speaking personally, my habit affected my self-esteem, and it affected the way I felt about my body. I felt like my life couldn't start until I figured this problem out.

This is suffering, and because of this suffering we keep searching for answers.

The search leads to a new diet to follow and initially, as we embrace the new program or diet that's going to help us curb our unwanted habit, our thinking quiets down. It seems like a solution to the problem we've been suffering with for so long. We have thoughts like, 'This is it. I have found the solution. If I just do these things, if I just follow these guidelines and these rules in this new program, everything's going to be great, and my suffering is going to be reduced.'

As a result, temporarily, our thinking about the unwanted overeating habit settles down. And like I say, for the first two or three days or a week, that reduction in the amount of thinking we've got about food is really helpful. We're able to stick to the program initially, specifically because our thinking has settled down.

However, as you and I both know, problems soon begin to arise.

Because we don't understand that we're living in the world of our thinking, not in the world of our circumstances, and because we don't understand the nature of thought—that it is like the weather, or like a river of energy flowing through us—our thinking begins to get stirred up again. Maybe we have a thought about bending the rules of the diet. Or maybe life gets turbulent (as it always does) and our thinking gets stirred up about that. Or we have a hard day and notice ourselves craving our favorite foods.

As we feel this happening, panic can set in. We don't want to fail again. We really wanted things to work out this time. So, we fight harder with our thinking, trying to get it and ourselves under control.

Now, that peaceful state that the new diet initiated has evaporated, and the quiet mind is gone. We're back to having very busy thinking, which is the problem we used food to solve in the first place. And unfortunately, we know exactly what will make that thinking stop: indulging in our favorite food or our unwanted overeating habit.

Having something 'forbidden' to eat does two important things (as we've discussed):

1. It temporarily shuts down all that thinking, all that arguing that's going on within you. It quiets all the chatter, if only for a moment.

2. It is the valve that releases some of the pressure you feel from all that thinking.

. . .

This experience became a cycle I was trapped in for years. Unfortunately, when we don't understand the nature of thought, and when our latest diet does actually work for a few days or weeks, those releases can look like an answer. Sadly, when our thinking gets stirred up again, we can feel like we've failed. I know I did. Every single time. I felt like I just didn't have enough willpower or discipline to make a diet stick.

However, what's really going on is that the whole diet premise is flawed. As you've hopefully begun to see, when we begin to understand how our thinking works, the need for diets falls away. When I stopped looking toward what I perceived was 'broken' within me (cravings) and began to look toward my innate health—and began to see my cravings for the wisdom-bearing entities they are—that's when my overeating habit began to resolve itself. I didn't need someone outside myself to tell me how to manage my food intake. What I needed was someone to show me that I was never broken in the first place.

# Chapter 19

## *Coffee and Weed*

I was in a coffee shop the other day and overheard the two guys behind me in line discussing how much coffee they drank on any given day. One of them said this: "I have five or six cups of coffee every day. If I don't have enough coffee, I smoke too many joints."

His comment made me smile to myself because, in a surprising way, it also pointed to something important about the understanding I'm sharing in this book.

We've probably all experienced what I call 'habit shifting,' where we force ourselves to give up one habit only to have another one take its place. We stop overeating only to take up smoking. We give up smoking only to spend an excessive amount of time playing video games. Habit shifting can look like a problem, but really, it's another example of our perfect design. It points to the metaphor I used earlier about the Instant Pot. We need our unwanted habits; they are the pressure release valve in our design. So, when we try to remove that valve by forcing ourselves to give up an unwanted habit, it simply pops up in a different location because it has to exist somewhere.

When this happens, we can begin to think of ourselves as having 'addictive personalities' and blame ourselves for a perceived lack of self-discipline or willpower. But what if this phenomenon was actually proving that your human design is kind and perfect?

Cravings will continue to speak to you until you hear what they have to say. They will never give up on you. Remember, they are trying to remind you that your natural state of being is one of calm, quiet wisdom. They are trying to let you know that you're caught up in Nancy's world rather than being connected with your true, wise, calm state of being. But if you use willpower to force yourself to live without an unwanted habit, another one is going to appear somewhere else in your life.

Habit shifting is not an indication of how broken we can be; it is actually proof of how whole we are.

# Chapter 20

## *Walking Barefoot*

The other day I had some pain in one of my big toes and, coincidentally, when I was next on YouTube, I was shown some videos about barefoot shoes. If you're not familiar, barefoot shoes are designed without all the padding and support we normally associate with running shoes. Instead, they try to mimic as closely as possible the experience of walking barefoot. The shoes are wide at the front to give toes the space to spread out, and they have a very thin sole. Proponents say that wearing this type of foot gear is better for our feet and our posture, and corrects things like bunions. However, most of them advised changing to these types of shoes gradually and carefully: the hosts of several of the videos I watched mentioned that when they switched from conventional shoes to barefoot shoes, they did so over a long period of time in order to avoid injury and excessive discomfort.

I advise this cautious approach to what I've been teaching you here as well: when we switch to an entirely new and also perhaps unconventional way of doing something, a few different things are going to happen:

1. We're going to experience some push-back, both from ourselves and from others.

In the case of the barefoot shoes, some of them look like foot gloves; they've got a separate compartment for each toe. If you're ever starved for attention, walk around in a pair of those for an hour or two—you'll receive endless questions and possibly also speculation about your sanity.

2. We could injure ourselves if we go too far, too fast. Sometimes change is longer lasting if it happens slowly. People who sell you shoes have known this for eons—we break in our new hiking boots before doing the Appalachian Trail, and we wouldn't dream of wearing a new pair of heels to an all-day meeting.

Diet culture doesn't believe in this, of course. I'm sure that, like me, you've sometimes tried to change the way you're eating overnight when you've stumbled across a diet or program that promised miraculous results. Speaking personally, that kind of change never worked for me, not least because it was unreasonable to expect myself to adapt to such drastic measures instantaneously.

I bring this up in order to help you manage your expectations about change when it comes to learning the secret language of cravings. This is not a 'lose 30 pounds in 30 days' type of approach. If it's not obvious yet, the understanding you've just explored in this book is about more than food, more than eating— and more than the secret language of cravings. It's about your true nature and how brilliant and beautiful that is. It's about the perfection behind our human design and how that design is always working for us, not against us. It's about how we are always healthy, always whole, even when we are struggling with something like an overeating problem, and how that 'problem' is itself pointing us back to our innate wholeness and well-being.

The secret language of cravings is a language of love and of wisdom. When we see it for what it is, every aspect of our life is changed and sweetened. Life becomes a joyful, gentle exploration rather than a journey filled with disheartening trials and challenges. Trials and challenges are part of life, of course, but they have less weight when we view them knowing we are all infinitely resilient and that we can rely on the well of peace that is always at our core, and always available to us.

My wish for you is that this book is the beginning of your exploration into all that you are. I also hope that you can remember, as often as possible, that your food cravings are not a problem. When we see them as the wise messages they really are, we begin to see that they are a gift. And that they are whispering, "You are well. You are whole. You are love."

# Find Freedom From Overeating

To continue your exploration and understanding of the secret language of cravings, I've created a complimentary starter kit for readers of this book. The kit includes:

1. A video tutorial outlining the free resources I offer to assist those looking to resolve an overeating habit, as well as tips for the next steps you can take in order to deepen your exploration of the inside-out understanding.

2. A complimentary copy of my book *An Introduction to the Three Principles* to help you expand your understanding of this psychological paradigm of health.

3. Complimentary access to my five-part video course, *How to Hack Your Thinking and Let Go of Unwanted Habits*, which will reinforce what you've learned in this book.

4. A complimentary subscription to my twice-monthly newsletter so that you'll receive all my special

subscriber-only offers about the upcoming resources, education, and support I'm offering for those looking to resolve an unwanted overeating habit.

To receive your complimentary copy of
this starter kit go to:
AlexandraAmor.com/starterkit

# About the Author

Alexandra Amor is a lifelong explorer of what it means to be human.

For over 15 years Alexandra has been writing both fiction and non-fiction books, all with the themes of love, connection, and the search for understanding. She began her writing career with an Amazon best-selling, award-winning memoir about ten years she spent in a cult in the 1990s.

Alexandra lives in a magical fishing village on Vancouver Island and spends each day writing, podcasting, exploring the inside-out understanding, and creating. When she's not doing that you'll likely find her walking on a local beach or worrying that the vacuum cleaner feels ignored. In her spare time she serves on the boards of her local hospice association and local seniors' independent living facility.

Learn more at AlexandraAmor.com

# Also by Alexandra Amor

### Non-fiction

It's Not About the Food: A Revolutionary Approach For Those Who Have Tried Everything To Heal The Drive To Overeat

Cult, A Love Story: Ten Years Inside a Canadian Cult and the Subsequent Long Road of Recovery

### A Town Called Horse Mysteries

Horse With No Name

A Town Called Horse: 4 historical mystery novellas

### Freddie Lark Mystery

Lark Underground

### Juliet Island Romantic Mystery

Love and Death at the Inn

# Acknowledgments

Huge thanks to copyeditor Jennifer McIntyre whose brilliant editing work and incisive, always valuable feedback makes every book I write far better than I could ever manage alone. Jen, you are worth your weight in gold and I am so grateful for our working relationship!

Thanks also to the Tuesday mastermind group. You inspire me and remind me to keep looking toward wisdom for answers. I love you all.

# Notes

## 6. Why Everything You've Tried Hasn't Worked

1.  https://www.nationalforests.org/blog/underground-mycor
    rhizal-network

## 11. Insight and Wisdom

1.  Gilbert, Elizabeth Eat, Pray, Love p16
2.  Gilbert, Elizabeth Eat, Pray, Love p16
3.  Gilbert, Elizabeth Eat, Pray, Love p16

Made in the USA
Coppell, TX
02 February 2024

28530047R00069